No Salt Recipes

Your GO-TO Cookbook of Healthy, Low-Sodium Ideas!

Table of Contents

Introduction 4

No Salt Added Breakfast Recipes…................................... 6

    1 – Honey and Yogurt Fruit Cups 7

    2 – Carrot and Oatmeal Muffins 9

    3 – Cranberry and Sweet Potato Doughnuts 12

    4 – Low Sodium Home Fries 15

    5 – Blueberry-Pear Granola 17

No Salt Added Lunch, Dinner, Appetizer and Side Dish Recipes… 19

    6 – Cranberry Pineapple Chicken 20

    7 – Lemon-Kissed Salmon 22

    8 – Mushroom and Barley Soup 25

    9 – Roast Tenderloin 27

    10 – Slow Cooked Lime Chicken 29

    11 – Roasted Halibut 31

    12 – Turkey Spaghetti Squash 33

    13 – Ginger and Honey Crusted Chicken 36

    14 – Leek and Potato Soup 38

    15 – Vegetables and Sole 40

    16 – Herbed Apples and Pork 43

    17 – Sesame Chicken Salad 46

    18 – Potato and Lentil Soup 48

19 – Pepper and Walnut Pasta 51

20 – Chicken, Asparagus and Pasta................................... 54

21 – Spicy Jambalaya 57

22 – Cauliflower Soup 60

23 – Bean Rice Bowl... 62

24 – Pork Chops and Fruit Salsa.. 64

25 – Apple Pecan Salad 67

No Salt and Low Salt Dessert Recipes... 70

26 – Balsamic Grilled Pineapples 71

27 – Banana Peanut Butter Muffins 73

28 – Mango Sorbet... 76

29 – Quick Apple Phyllo Pie.. 78

30 – Raspberry Pears 81

Conclusion 83

Introduction

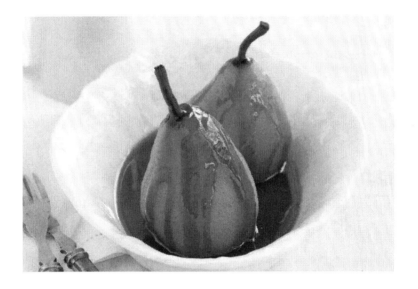

Have you ever tried to cut back on your sodium intake?

Can this be done using prepared foods? Usually not.

Can you make no salt added meals at home that are tasty? Yes, you can!

Your nutritionist or physician usually provides you with safe foods lists that you can take with you when you shop for groceries. Be sure to read the labels on canned and prepared foods.

Select frozen or fresh veggies and fruits to give you added control over your salt intake. Eliminate as many salty foods as you can from your diet and use less salt when you cook.

Choose foods listed as low sodium but check the labels to be sure. Low sodium foods should have not much more than 140 mg sodium for each serving.

Eating meals cooked at home is an excellent way to lower your intake of salt. When you make dishes yourself, you know just how much salt they contain. Using recipes like the delicious ones in this cookbook makes it easier to stick to a no salt added diet.

Think outside the box and cook creatively. Season your dishes with pepper, vinegar, ginger, garlic, lemon and spices and herbs. You don't have to sacrifice taste to stick to a no salt added diet!

No Salt Added Breakfast Recipes...

1 – Honey and Yogurt Fruit Cups

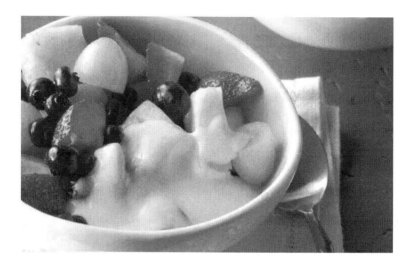

You'll look forward to eating breakfast when it is this appealing and tasty. The combination of yogurt and fresh fruit always disappears quickly in my home.

Makes 6 Servings

Cooking + Prep Time: 15 minutes

Ingredients:

- 4 1/2 cups of fresh fruit, cubed or chunked – grapes, bananas, apples pears are good
- 6 oz. of yogurt – lemon, mandarin orange or vanilla
- 1 tbsp. of honey, organic

- 1/2 tsp. of orange zest, grated
- 1/4 tsp. of almond extract, pure

Instructions:

1. Divide the fruit in six separate bowls for serving.

2. Combine extract, zest, honey and yogurt. Spoon this over your fruit. Serve.

2 – Carrot and Oatmeal Muffins

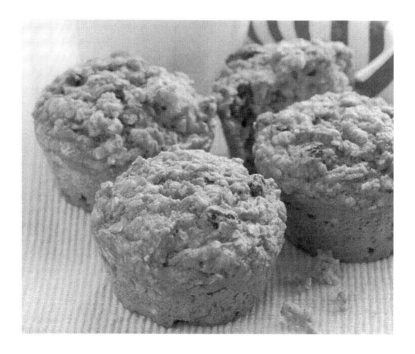

This is not a coffee shop muffin. It's low sodium and healthy. The taste is light and delicious, with cinnamon and a sweet carrot tinge. If you like, you can lightly toast these muffins and enjoy them with a bit of light cream cheese.

Makes 6 Servings

Cooking + Prep Time: 35 minutes

Ingredients:

- 1 egg, medium
- 2 tsp. of oil, canola
- 1/2 cup of Stevia®
- 2 tbsp. of yogurt, non-fat
- 1/2 tsp. of vanilla extract, pure
- 1 cup of flour, all-purpose
- 1/2 cup of flour, whole wheat
- 1/4 tsp. of salt substitute
- 1/4 tsp. of baking soda
- 1 tsp. of baking powder
- 1/2 tsp. of cinnamon, ground
- 1/4 tsp. of nutmeg, ground
- 1 cup of peeled, shredded carrots
- 1/4 cup of oatmeal, not instant type
- 1/2 cup of buttermilk, low fat

Instructions:

1. Preheat the oven to 375F.

2. Separate egg into yolk and white. Set yolk aside. Whisk the white till it becomes frothy. Add oil. Whisk till mixture is smooth. Add Stevia®, vanilla extract, egg yolk and yogurt.

3. Whisk new mixture till it is smooth.

4. Place both flours, salt substitute, nutmeg, cinnamon, baking soda and baking powder in sifter. Sift into mixing bowl. Sprinkle oatmeal flakes on top.

5. Fold creamed mixture into flour mixture. Add carrot shreds slowly as you blend the mixtures.

6. Add buttermilk and blend just till smooth.

7. Line muffin tin with papers. Fill them with batter. Bake for 10-15 minutes. Serve.

3 – Cranberry and Sweet Potato Doughnuts

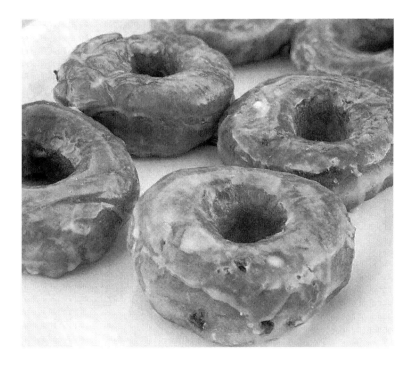

This is a breakfast take on "spudnuts", or doughnuts made with mashed potatoes. Not surprisingly, that recipe originated in Idaho. It has been reworked into this recipe that uses cranberries and sweet potatoes for a unique and delightful breakfast.

Makes 2 dozen doughnuts

Cooking + Prep Time: 1 hour 5 minutes plus rising time

Ingredients:

- 1/4 cup of sugar, granulated
- 1 1/2 tsp. of yeast, dry active
- 1 tsp. of cinnamon, ground
- 1/2 tsp. of salt substitute
- 4 cups of flour, all-purpose
- 1 cup of milk, 2%
- 1/4 cup of shortening
- 2 tbsp. of water, filtered
- 2 eggs, medium
- 1/2 cup of sweet potatoes, mashed
- 1/2 cup of dried cranberries, chopped finely
- **To fry:** oil
- 1 cup of sugar, powdered
- 2-3 tbsp. of apple juice or cider

Instructions:

1. Combine 1 1/2 cup of flour with salt substitute, cinnamon, yeast and sugar in large sized bowl.

2. In small sized pan, heat water, milk and shortening till temp is 120 to 130F. Add this mixture to the dry ingredients.

3. Beat at med. speed for two minutes. Add cranberries, eggs and mashed potatoes. Beat for two more minutes. Add enough flour to form firm dough. Don't knead the dough.

4. Place dough in greased bowl and turn one time to grease top. Cover. Allow to sit in warm area of home for an hour or so, till it doubles.

5. Punch the dough down. Place on floured cutting board. Roll to 1/2" in thickness.

6. Use doughnut cutter to cut and reroll scraps to use all dough. Place on greased cookie sheets with one inch between them. Cover. Allow to rise till it doubles. This will take about a half hour.

7. In deep fryer or electric skillet, heat the oil up to 375F. Fry the doughnuts, several at a time, till both sides are a golden brown color. Drain them on paper towels.

8. Combine the apple juice or cider with powdered sugar. Dip the warm doughnuts in this glaze. Serve.

4 – Low Sodium Home Fries

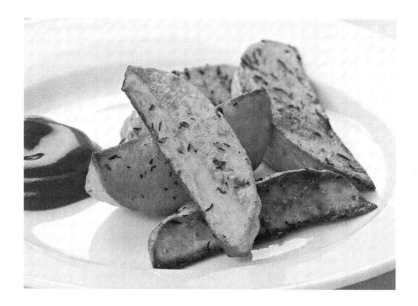

This recipe uses spray-type olive oil to enhance its overall consistency. The onions are lightly caramelized and the precooked potatoes make some delicious home fries.

Makes 2 Servings

Cooking + Prep Time: 40 minutes

Ingredients:

- 8 oz. of diced potatoes
- Oil spray
- 1 diced onion, small

- 1/8 tsp. of salt substitute
- Pepper, black, ground

Instructions:

1. Place diced potatoes in glass bowl in microwave. Cook for a minute on high setting. Stir potatoes and allow them to rest.

2. Place non-stick, large sized skillet on med-high. Spray with oil lightly. Add onions when pan becomes hot. Toss frequently while cooking till onions start turning light brown in color.

3. As onions cook, repeat first step with potatoes two more times. Allow them to rest between periods of cooking.

4. When onions are brown, add potatoes, salt substitute and ground pepper to pan. Lightly spray with oil once more. Toss home fries till potatoes are browned lightly. Serve.

5 – Blueberry-Pear Granola

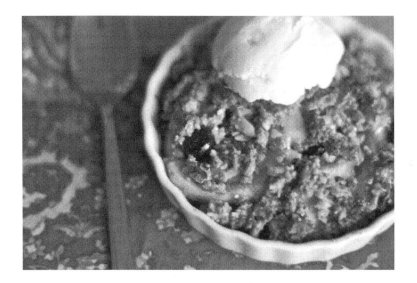

If you love oatmeal, you'll fall in love with this dish, too. The granola, pears and blueberries make a wonderful breakfast – if you add ice cream, they can be served as a dessert! They are THAT good.

Makes 10 Servings

Cooking + Prep Time: 10 minutes plus 3 to 4 hours slow cooker time

Ingredients:

- 5 peeled, sliced pears, medium
- 2 cups of blueberries, unsweetened, frozen or fresh

- 1/2 cup of sugar, brown, packed
- 1/3 cup of apple juice, unsweetened
- 1 tbsp. of flour, all-purpose
- 1 tbsp. of lemon juice, fresh if possible
- 2 tsp. of cinnamon, ground
- 2 tbsp. of butter, unsalted
- 3 cups of granola with no raisins

Instructions:

1. Combine first 7 ingredients in slow cooker. Add a bit of butter. Sprinkle the granola over the top.

2. Cover slow cooker. Cook on the low setting for three to four hours, till fruit has become tender. Serve.

No Salt Added Lunch, Dinner, Appetizer and Side Dish Recipes...

6 – Cranberry Pineapple Chicken

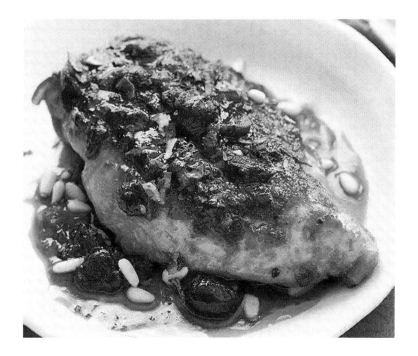

This poultry dish will tantalize the tongues of even the finickiest of eaters, including kids. The pineapples and cranberries give chicken new life.

Makes 8 Servings

Cooking + Prep Time: 55 minutes

Ingredients:

- 4 lbs. of halved chicken breast, boneless, skinless
- 1 x 16-oz. can of cranberry sauce, whole
- 1 x 20-oz. can of drained pineapple, crushed
- 1/2 tsp. of cinnamon, ground

Instructions:

1. Preheat the oven to 375F.

2. Place the chicken in 13x9", lightly greased baking dish. Pierce with fork.

3. Layer the pineapple and cranberry sauce over the chicken. Sprinkle cinnamon on top.

4. Cover the dish. Bake in 375F oven for 20-25 minutes. Remove the cover. Bake for 15 minutes more, till chicken has cooked completely through. Serve hot.

7 – Lemon-Kissed Salmon

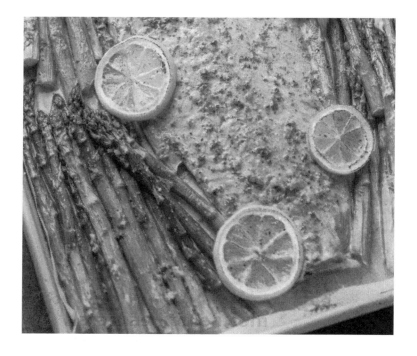

Salmon is one of the best sources of protein in meals. Protein is vital, since it triggers you to feel full. Your body also needs protein to build and maintain healthy muscles. In this recipe, lemon adds an extra touch of flavor to your salmon.

Makes 4 Servings

Cooking + Prep Time: 45 minutes

Ingredients:

- 4 x 5-oz. salmon fillets
- 2 tsp. + 2 tbsp. of oil, olive
- Salt substitute
- Pepper, black, ground
- 3 chopped tomatoes, ripe
- 2 shallots, chopped
- 2 tbsp. of lemon juice, fresh
- 1 tsp. of oregano, dried
- 1 tsp. of thyme, dried

Instructions:

1. Preheat oven to 400F.

2. Sprinkle the salmon fillets with 2 tsp. of oil, salt substitute and ground pepper. Stir shallots, tomatoes, 2 tbsp. oil, additional salt substitute, ground pepper, thyme, oregano and lemon juice in medium sized bowl and blend.

3. Place first salmon fillet with oiled side facing down, on foil sheet. Wrap foil ends to make a spiral. Spoon tomato mixture on salmon. Fold sides of foil over mixture and cover fully. Seal packet closed. Place foil packet on large cookie sheet.

4. Repeat till all salmon fillets are wrapped and set on cookie sheet.

5. Bake till salmon is barely cooked through, or about 20-25 minutes. Transfer packets to individual plates. Serve.

8 – Mushroom and Barley Soup

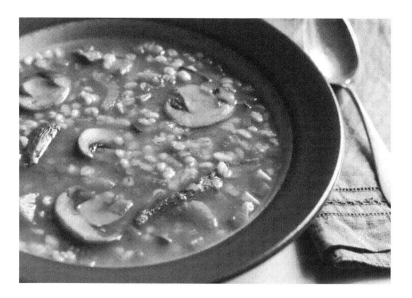

This is a soup I have always loved, but my old recipe took three hours. I needed something simpler, and here it is. It takes just about one hour. If you're a fan of this type of soup, you will fall hard for this recipe. It's so soothing on those cold nights of fall and winter.

Makes 6 Servings

Cooking + Prep Time: 1 hour 10 minutes

Ingredients:

- 1/4 cup of oil, olive
- 1 cup of onions, chopped
- 3/4 cup of carrots, diced
- 1/2 cup of celery, chopped
- 1 tsp. of garlic, minced
- 1 lb. of sliced mushrooms, fresh
- 6 cups of broth, chicken, low sodium
- 3/4 cup of barley
- Salt substitute and ground pepper, as desired

Instructions:

1. Heat oil in large sized pot on med. heat.

2. Add garlic, celery, carrots and onions. Stir while cooking till onions become transparent and tender. Add mushrooms and stir. Continue cooking for several minutes.

3. Add chicken broth to mixture, then barley. Bring to boil. Reduce the heat down to low. Cover pot. Simmer till barley becomes tender, or 45-50 minutes. Season as desired and serve.

9 – Roast Tenderloin

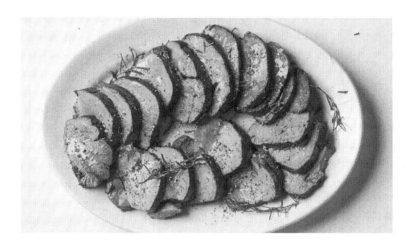

Tenderloin is a positive choice in meat for no salt added diets, since it doesn't have a lot of sodium in it. Tender cuts are the best, being low in fat with a milder flavor than some other meats. Since you're not going to add salt, you'll use other ingredients to add zest to the meal.

Makes 8-10 Servings

Cooking + Prep Time: 50 minutes

Ingredients:

- 1 beef tenderloin, whole, with visible fat trimmed off
- Salt substitute
- 2 tsp. of sugar, granulated

- 1/2 cup of crushed peppercorns, tri-color
- 1 stick of butter, unsalted
- 2 crushed garlic cloves

Instructions:

1. Preheat oven to 475F.

2. Place tenderloin on roasting rack. Sprinkle with sugar and salt substitute to deepen the meat's flavors.

3. Press peppercorns over entire meat surface. Insert meat thermometer. Place tenderloin in oven till temp is 120-125F. This is medium rare to rare. Adjust to your preferred level of doneness.

4. As meat roasts, melt garlic in butter in small sized skillet. Allow butter to brown a bit. Remove and discard garlic.

5. Remove meat when done. Pour garlic butter atop meat gently – don't worry if it sizzles; this is normal.

6. Use foil to cover meat loosely. Allow it to rest for 8-10 minutes. Slice and serve.

10 – Slow Cooked Lime Chicken

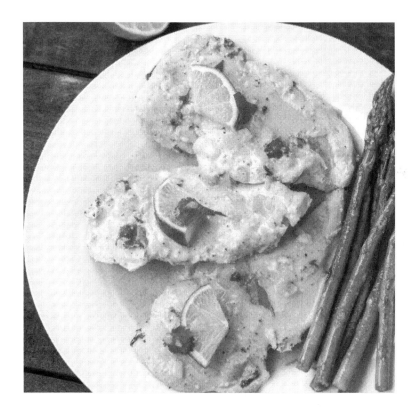

This dish will please the whole family, or a table of guests, and the prep work is minimal. Just get the ingredients ready to go and let the slow cooker do the work. The lime adds to the taste of the chicken and **Makes** the dish unique.

Makes 4 Servings

Cooking + Prep Time: 15 minutes + 8-10 hours slow cooker time

Ingredients:

- 1 1/4 lbs. of halved chicken breast, boneless, skinless
- 1/3 cup of lime juice, fresh if available
- 2 cups of chicken broth, low sodium
- 1 minced garlic clove
- 1/2 tsp. of thyme leaves, dried
- 1/4 tsp. of pepper, black, ground
- 2 tbsp. of butter, unsalted
- 2 cups of instant rice, uncooked

Instructions:

1. Place chicken in slow cooker. Add stock and lime juice. Add butter, pepper, thyme and garlic.

2. Cover slow cooker. Cook on the low setting till chicken becomes quite tender. This usually takes eight to 10 hours. In last 15 minutes cooking, stir in rice to cook. Mix well and serve.

11 – Roasted Halibut

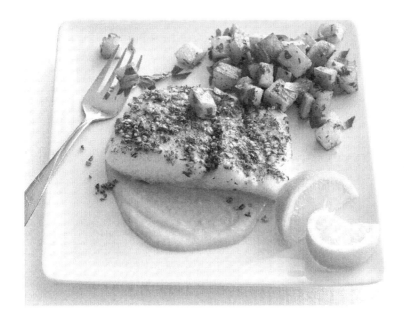

Using just six ingredients, this is a simple no salt added dish. The mixed berries provide the dish with a tangy zip and enhance the taste of the halibut.

Makes 4 Servings

Cooking + Prep Time: 1/2 hour

Ingredients:

- 4 oz. of halibut
- Non-stick spray

- 2 tbsp. of margarine, unsalted, melted and cooled
- 3/4 cup of hazelnuts, chopped finely
- 1 cup of mixed berries, frozen, thawed
- 1/2 tsp. of sugar, granulated

Instructions:

1. Preheat the oven to 400F. Spray 10x15x1" baking pan using non-stick spray and set it aside.

2. Rinse the halibut fillets and pat them dry using paper towels.

3. Place margarine in shallow dish. Place hazelnuts in separate shallow dish. Dip the halibut in margarine first and coat both sides of each fillet with margarine and nuts. Place the fillets on pre-sprayed pan.

4. Bake for eight to 10 minutes, till fish will flake when you use a fork to test it.

5. As fish roasts, puree berries in food processor. Pour pureed berries through strainer and remove seeds. Stir sugar into the strained sauce.

6. When fish is done, serve with chilled or warmed berry sauce.

12 – Turkey Spaghetti Squash

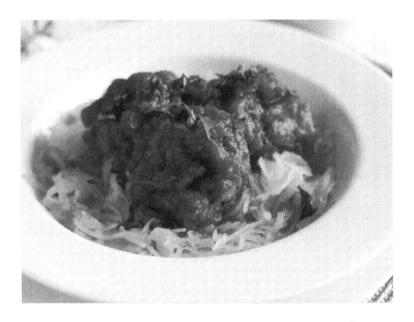

This unique, no salt added dish puts regular types of pasta to shame. I always plan to have leftovers and we almost NEVER do – that's how good it is!

Makes 6 Servings

Cooking + Prep Time: 2 hours and 10 minutes

Ingredients:

- 1 halved, de-seeded spaghetti squash, small
- 1 tbsp. of oil, olive

- 1/2 cup of onion, minced
- 3 minced garlic cloves
- 2 minced green onions
- 12 oz. of turkey, white meat, ground
- 2 cups of tomatoes, crushed
- 2 tbsp. of wine, red
- 2 tsp. of capers
- 2 tsp. of oregano, fresh, minced
- 2 tsp. of pepper flakes, red, crushed
- 2 tsp. of chopped parsley, fresh

Instructions:

1. Preheat the oven to 350F.

2. Place both squash halves with the cut side facing down on baking sheet. Leave uncovered and bake for 40-60 minutes. Fork should easily go into shell. Allow squash to cool. Scoop strands out. Set them aside.

3. Heat oil in large skillet on med-high. Add green onions, onions and garlic. Sauté for two to three minutes. Add turkey. Cook for three to four minutes. Add wine and tomatoes. Bring to boil. Then reduce heat. Simmer for 18-20 minutes.

4. Add parsley, pepper flakes, oregano and capers to pot. Simmer for four to five minutes. Top squash with sauce. Serve.

13 – Ginger and Honey Crusted Chicken

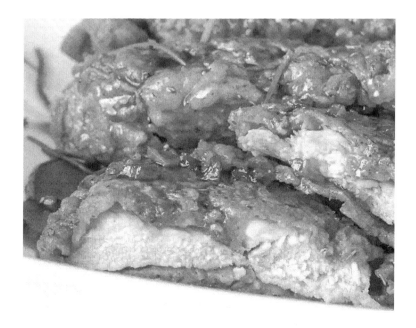

Ginger, honey and orange juice give this chicken a taste like fried chicken, but it's not fried, so it's healthier. The chicken stays crispy, with low calories and low fat, too.

Makes 4 Servings

Cooking + Prep Time: 35 minutes

- 4 halved small chicken breasts, boneless, skinless
- Non-stick spray
- 1 tbsp. of honey, pure
- 1 tbsp. of orange juice, fresh if available
- 1/4 tsp. of ginger, ground
- 1/4 tsp. of pepper, black, ground
- 1/3 cup of crushed corn flakes
- 1/2 tsp. of parsley flakes, dried

Instructions:

1. Spray shallow baking pan using cooking spray. Place chicken in this pan.

2. Combine ginger, orange juice, honey and ground pepper together in small sized bowl.

3. Brush honey mixture on the chicken.

4. Combine parsley and corn flakes. Sprinkle mixture over the chicken, coating it.

5. Leave uncovered and bake at 350F for 17-20 minutes. Chicken should be tender, with no pink anymore. Remove from oven and serve hot.

14 – Leek and Potato Soup

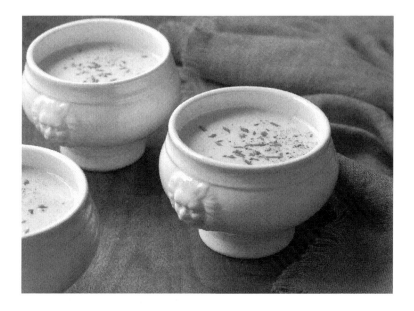

This creamy, low sodium soup has a wonderful taste from the leeks. It goes great with bread. You can heat it up the next day for an extra treat.

Makes 8 Servings

Cooking + Prep Time: 1 1/2 hour

Ingredients:

- 1 cup of butter, unsalted
- 2 sliced leeks
- Salt substitute and ground pepper, as desired

- 1 quart of chicken broth, low sodium
- 1 tbsp. of corn starch
- 4 cups of peeled, diced potatoes
- 2 cups of cream, heavy

Instructions:

1. Melt the butter in large sized pot on med. heat. Cook the leeks in the butter and season as desired, frequently stirring till tender. This usually takes 12-15 minutes.

2. Stir the corn starch into chicken broth. Pour the broth into the large pot. Add potatoes. Bring mixture to boil. Season as desired.

3. Add cream and reduce heat. Simmer for 1/2 hour or longer, till potatoes become tender. Season as desired and serve.

15 – Vegetables and Sole

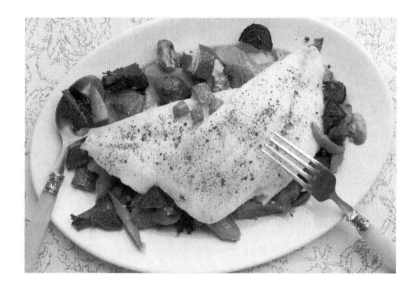

The veggies and fish fillet in this dish offer you protein and fiber, and the calorie and sodium counts are still low. It is made and served in parchment paper packets, so it's super easy to clean up, too.

Makes 4 Servings

Cooking + Prep Time: 50 minutes

Ingredients:

- 4 oz. of skinless sole fillets, frozen or fresh
- 8 oz. of trimmed green beans, thin, fresh
- 2 de-seeded, sliced medium sweet peppers, red

- 1 wedge-cut onion, small
- 1/4 to 1/2 tsp. of red pepper, crushed
- 4 sliced garlic cloves
- 2 tsp. of oil, canola
- 1 1/2 tsp. of lemon peel, shredded finely

Instructions:

1. Preheat the oven to 400F. If you're using frozen sole, thaw it. Rinse it and pat it dry using paper towels. Set fish aside.

2. Cut four x 12x20-inch parchment paper pieces. Fold them in half crossways. Crease them. Unfold them and lay them flat.

3. On 1/2 of each piece of parchment paper, arrange the onion, beans and sweet peppers. Sprinkle them with garlic and crushed pepper. Top them with pieces of sole. Use oil to drizzle and sprinkle the top with the lemon peel.

4. To prepare the packets, fold the paper over the veggies and sole. To seal them, fold each open side over one-half inch. Fold over one-half inch again.

5. Place the packets on large cookie sheet. Bake for 15 minutes or so, till sole flakes readily when you test it using

a fork. Open packets carefully and check for doneness. Serve.

16 – Herbed Apples and Pork

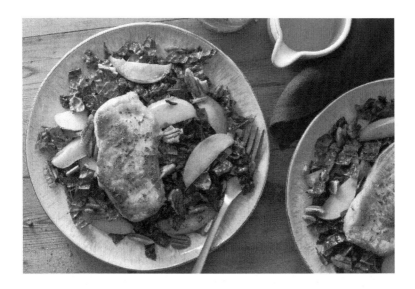

When I serve these apples with pork to guests, I am almost always asked for this recipe. You can make it with pork tenderloin as well – it will still come out tasty.

Makes 14 Servings

Cooking + Prep Time: 3 hours 45 minutes plus 6-8 hours refrigerator time

Ingredients:

- 1 tsp. dried each of sage, thyme, rosemary and marjoram
- Salt substitute and ground black pepper, as desired

- 6 lb. roast, pork loin
- 4 cored, peeled, chunk-cut apples, tart
- 1 chopped onion, red
- 3 tbsp. of sugar, brown
- 1 cup of juice, apple
- 2/3 cup of maple syrup, real

Instructions:

1. Combine salt substitute, ground pepper, marjoram, thyme and sage in small sized bowl. Rub the mixture over the roast.

2. Cover. Refrigerate the roast for six to eight hours. You can just leave it in overnight, if you like.

3. Preheat the oven to 325F.

4. Remove roast from fridge and place in shallow roasting pan. Bake at 325F for 1-1 1/2 hours. Drain the fat away.

5. Mix brown sugar, onion and apples in medium sized bowl. Spoon this around the roast. Continue cooking for another hour. Internal temp of roast should be 145F.

6. Transfer roast and fixings to serving platter. Keep food warm.

7. To prepare gravy, skim the excess fat from the meat juices. Pour the drippings into a skillet. Add and stir syrup and apple juice.

8. Stir and cook on med-high heat till liquid is reduced by 1/2. Slice roast. Serve with the gravy.

17 – Sesame Chicken Salad

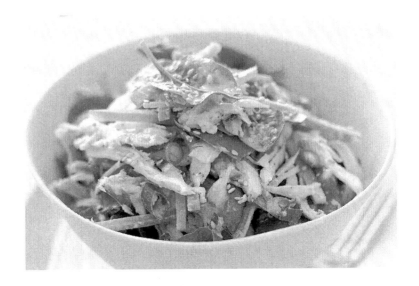

This is a recipe based on European style salad dishes. It uses mixed chicken strips, green onions, radishes and baby corn. After you toss it with the sesame oil and vinegar dressing, it's a dream of a meal, and has no salt added.

Makes 6 Servings

Cooking + Prep Time: 25 minutes

Ingredients:

- 1 x 10-oz. pkg. of Italian or European style salad greens, torn
- 2 cups of cooked chicken, chopped or shredded

- 1 x 8 3/4 oz. can of drained, halved crossways baby corn
- 2 sliced green onions
- 1/4 cup of radishes, sliced
- 1/2 cup of orange juice, fresh if available
- 1/4 cup of vinegar, white or rice
- 1/2 tsp. of sesame oil, toasted
- 1/4 tsp. of pepper, black, ground
- 1 1/2 tsp. of toasted sesame seeds

Instructions:

1. Combine salad greens, radishes, green onions, baby corn and chicken in large sized bowl.

2. To prepare dressing, combine orange juice, pepper, sesame oil and vinegar in a jar with a screw-top lid. Cover. Shake it well.

3. Pour the dressing over the greens. Gently toss to coat greens. Divide the greens mixture in six bowls. Sprinkle with the sesame seeds and serve.

18 – Potato and Lentil Soup

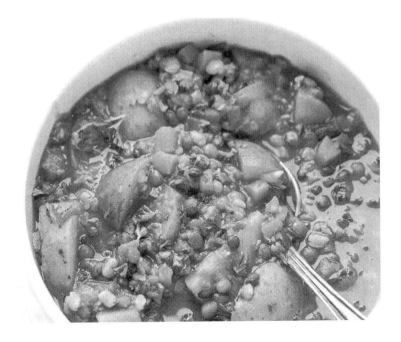

This is such a simple soup that you may be surprised at the delicious taste. It has a delectable thickness and tastes great served with low sodium sourdough bread.

Makes 12 Servings

Cooking + Prep Time: 1 1/4 hour

Ingredients:

- 2 tbsp. of butter, unsalted
- 1 chopped large onion, sweet

- 4 stalks of chopped celery
- 4 chopped medium potatoes, red
- 1 chopped carrot
- 3 garlic cloves
- 1/4 tsp. each of ground allspice, cumin seeds and cayenne pepper
- 1/8 tsp. of cloves, ground
- A dash of pepper, black, ground
- 1 qt. of broth, vegetable, low sodium
- 1 1/2 cups of red lentils, dry
- 2 cups of water, filtered
- 1 cup of kale, chopped roughly
- 1/4 cup of chopped cilantro, fresh

Instructions:

1. Melt butter in large sized sauce pan on med. heat. Add celery and onion and stir. Cook till they are tender. Add garlic, potatoes and carrot and mix.

2. Continue cooking and stirring for five minutes or so, till butter has coated potatoes well. Season using ground pepper, cloves, cayenne pepper, cumin and allspice.

3. Add veggie broth. Mix in lentils. Add as much water as you need to cover all the ingredients.

4. Bring to boil, then reduce heat. Add kale and stir. Cook and stir occasionally for 30-40 minutes, till lentils have become tender. Add cilantro and mix. Continue to cook for four to six minutes, until the thickness is as you desire. Serve.

19 – Pepper and Walnut Pasta

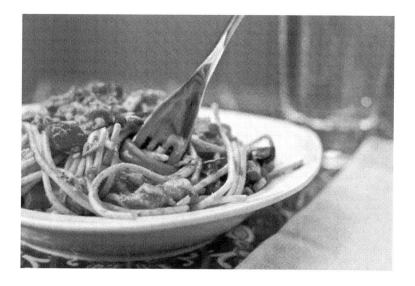

This veggie pasta dish only takes 30 minutes to put together, and the parsley and rosemary add flavor without added salt. The recipe is packed with fiber and antioxidants, too, so it will keep you feeling full.

Makes 4 Servings

Cooking + Prep Time: 1/2 hour

Ingredients:

- 6 oz. of whole grain pasta
- 1 tbsp. of oil, olive
- 1/4 cup of chopped walnuts

- 4 sliced garlic cloves, large
- 2 de-seeded, sliced bite-sized lengthways medium sweet peppers, green or red
- 1 wedge-cut small onion, red
- 1 cup of cherry tomatoes, halved
- 1/4 cup of parsley, snipped
- 1/2 tsp. of crushed rosemary, dried
- 1/4 tsp. of pepper, black, ground

Instructions:

1. Cook the pasta using the instructions on the package. Drain it and set it aside.

2. Heat oil on med. in large sized skillet. Add garlic and walnuts. Cook for a couple minutes and stir frequently till they are light brown.

3. Add onion and sweet peppers. Cook for five to seven minutes, till veggies are tender-crisp, still stirring.

4. Add the tomatoes. Stir while cooking till they have heated completely through. Add ground pepper, parsley and rosemary.

5. Pour pasta in large sized, shallow bowl. Top it with the pepper-walnut mixture. Gently toss and coat. Serve.

20 – Chicken, Asparagus and Pasta

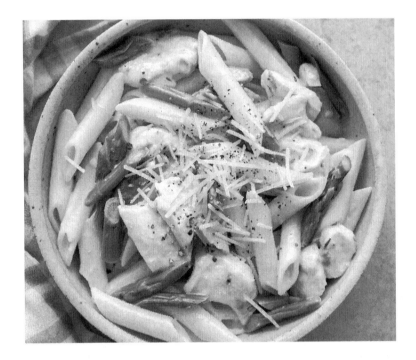

When you add the asparagus to the chicken and pasta in this dish, it turns an everyday no salt added recipe into a real treat. It's a light meal and is simple and quick to prepare – plus it tastes super!

Makes 8 Servings

Cooking + Prep Time: 40 minutes

- 1 x 16-oz. pkg. of penne pasta, dry
- 2 tbsp. of oil, olive
- 3/4 lb. of cubed chicken breast meat, boneless, skinless
- 4 minced garlic cloves
- 12 oz. of trimmed, 1" cut asparagus spears
- 1 tsp. of pepper flakes, crushed
- Salt substitute and ground black pepper, as desired
- 1/2 cup of Parmesan cheese, grated

Instructions:

1. Bring large sized pot of filtered water to boil. Cook the pasta using directions on package. Drain. Pour into medium bowl.

2. Heat 1 tbsp. of oil in large sized skillet on med. heat. Then sauté the chicken till firm but lightly browned. Remove chicken from the pan.

3. Add 1 tbsp. more oil to skillet. Stir while cooking pepper flakes, garlic and asparagus, till asparagus becomes tender. Add chicken. Cook for a couple minutes so flavors can blend. Season as desired.

4. Toss the pasta with asparagus and chicken mixture. Sprinkle Parmesan cheese over the top. Serve.

21 – Spicy Jambalaya

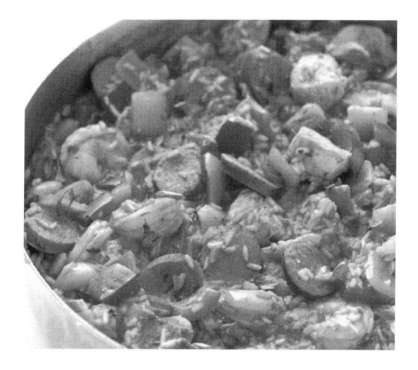

This is authentic jambalaya, since it uses the triad of Bayou ingredients – bell pepper, onion and celery. The rice, shrimp and lightly spicy sausage give it a truly distinctive taste. If you prefer a milder recipe, don't use any ground red pepper.

Makes 6 Servings

Cooking + Prep Time: 1 1/4 hour

Ingredients:

- 1 1/2 tsp. of oil, canola
- 6 oz. of chopped sausage, andouille
- 1 cup of onion, chopped
- 1 cup of bell pepper, green, chopped
- 1/2 cup of celery, chopped
- 5 minced cloves of garlic
- 2 cups of rice, whole-grain, cooked
- 1/2 tsp. of red pepper, ground
- 2 1/2 cups of broth, chicken, low sodium
- 1/2 tsp. of salt substitute
- 1 x 14 1/2 oz. can of undrained diced tomatoes, unsalted
- 12 oz. of peeled, de-veined shrimp, large
- 3 tbsp. of green onions, sliced

Instructions:

1. Heat large sized skillet on med-high. Add oil and swirl till it coats the pan. Add the sausage and sauté for three to five minutes, till it has browned.

2. Reduce the heat to med. Add celery, onion and bell pepper. Stir occasionally while cooking for seven to nine

minutes. Add the garlic and cook for a minute while constantly stirring.

3. Add red pepper and rice and stir frequently as you cook for a minute. Add tomatoes, broth and salt substitute and stir. Bring to boil. Cover skillet and reduce heat. Simmer for eight to 10 minutes, till liquid has been almost absorbed.

4. Add the shrimp by nestling them into the rice mixture. Cover. Simmer for three to five minutes, till shrimp are nearly done. Uncover skillet. Cook for three to five minutes more, till they are fully done. Remove skillet from heat. Sprinkle with the green onions and serve.

22 – Cauliflower Soup

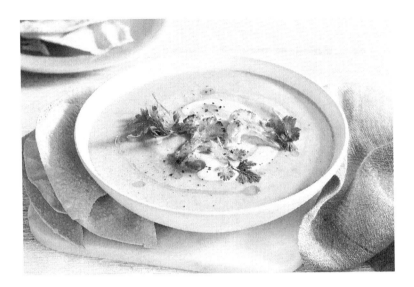

This cauliflower soup recipe has a creamy and smooth taste that many people think means it's fattening, but it's not. Your guests will be surprised at how low it is in sodium, and the few ingredients it uses.

Makes 6 Servings

Cooking + Prep Time: 1 3/4 hour

Ingredients:

- 2 floret-cut cauliflower heads
- Non-stick spray, olive oil flavored
- 1/4 cup of oil, olive

- 1 chopped onion, large
- 4 chopped garlic cloves
- 6 cups of water, filtered
- Salt substitute, as desired
- Pepper, black ground, as desired

Instructions:

1. Place cauliflower florets in large bowl of salted water. Let it stand for 15-20 minutes.

2. Drain cauliflower well. Arrange on foil sheet on cookie sheet. Spray evenly with olive oil flavored non-stick spray.

3. Preheat oven broiler. Set rack about six inches from heat source.

4. Broil cauliflower till browned. This usually takes 20-30 minutes.

5. Heat oil in large sized soup pot. Cook onion till it is translucent. Stir in roasted cauliflower and garlic.

6. Pour in water. Season as desired. Simmer till all veggies have become tender. This usually takes about a half-hour. Blend soup in pot with immersion blender till smooth and creamy. Serve.

23 – Bean Rice Bowl

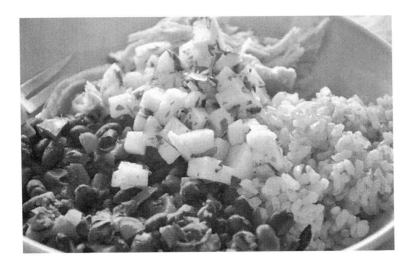

This is a hearty dish and packed with healthy protein, as well as being low in salt. It will leave you satisfied and full. You can make it ahead if you like and take it to school or to work.

Makes 1 Serving

Cooking + Prep Time: 15 minutes

Ingredients:

- 1 x 10 - 12-ounce pkg. of brown rice, pre-cooked, frozen
- 1/2 cup of rinsed, drained black beans
- 1/2 cup of salsa

- 2 tbsp. of cheddar cheese shreds
- 2 tbsp. of guacamole, store-bought
- Optional: hot sauce

Instructions:

1. Heat the rice using the directions on the package.

2. Combine salsa and beans in medium sized glass bowl. Cover partially. Cook at high power till the mixture has warmed all the way through. This usually only takes a minute or so.

3. Add 1 cup of rice and stir. Cover bowl. Cook till hot, or about one more minute. Top with the guacamole and cheese and add some hot sauce, as desired. Serve.

24 – Pork Chops and Fruit Salsa

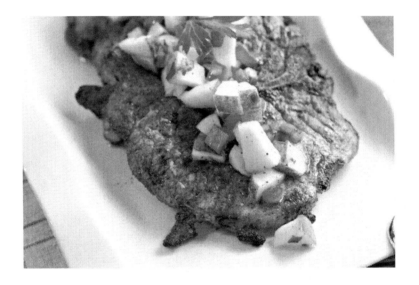

There are plenty of recipes that pair meat and salsa, but the salsa in THIS recipe is made from nectarines! It has a sunny, sweet taste. It goes especially well with grilled pork, and we serve this dish often in the summertime.

Makes 4 Servings

Cooking + Prep Time: 35 minutes

Ingredients:

- 2 pitted, diced nectarines, fresh
- 1 de-seeded, diced tomato, ripe
- 1/4 cup of onion, diced

- 2 tbsp. of chopped cilantro, fresh
- 1/4 tsp. +/- of pepper flakes, red, crushed
- 1 tsp. of chili powder
- 2 tbsp. of lime juice, fresh if available
- 1 tsp. of cumin, ground
- Salt substitute, as desired
- Pepper, black, ground, as desired
- 2 tbsp. of oil, olive
- 8 x 4-oz. pork chops, boneless

Instructions:

1. Preheat your grill for med-high. Oil grate lightly. Set four inches away from the heat.

2. Place pepper flakes, lime juice, cilantro, onion, tomato and nectarines in medium bowl. Toss and blend well.

3. Season as desired. Cover. Place in fridge for 1/2 hour so flavors have time to blend.

4. In small sized bowl, stir salt substitute, cumin, ground pepper and chili powder together.

5. Place oil in small sized bowl. Use oil to brush pork chops. Season on both sides with cumin mixture.

6. Lay pork chops on grill. Cook till browned lightly. This usually takes four to five minutes per side.

7. Place chops on individual plates. Top with salsa and serve.

25 – Apple Pecan Salad

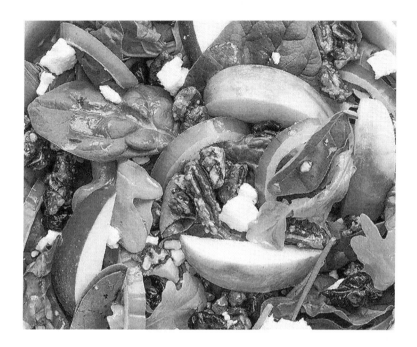

Apples are among the healthiest of fruits, and they add a filling element to this no salt added dish. The pecans give it a crunchy, sweet topping, along with heart healthy fats.

Makes 6 Servings

Cooking + Prep Time: 1 hour 5 minutes

Ingredients:

- Oil, olive
- 2 tbsp. of butter, unsalted

- 1/3 cup of brown sugar, light, packed
- 1 cup of halved pecans
- 1 fresh orange, juice + 3 tsp. of zest only
- 1 tsp. of mustard, Dijon
- 1 tbsp. of vinegar, white wine
- 3 tbsp. of oil, olive
- Salt substitute
- Pepper, black, fresh ground
- 2 cored, quartered, sliced green or red apples, medium
- 2 heads of endive, Belgian, separated in leaves
- 2 cups of greens, mixed, like arugula, etc.

Instructions:

1. Rub baking sheet lightly with oil and set it aside.

2. Heat large sized sauce pan on low heat. Add the sugar and butter. Simmer for several minutes and stir occasionally, till sugar dissolves completely and the color of the mixture has darkened.

3. Stir in the pecans gently till coated well. Transfer the nuts to baking sheet and separate into a single layer. Allow them to cool so the caramel will harden.

4. Combine the orange juice, orange zest, oil, vinegar and mustard in large sized salad bowl. Use a whisk to stir thoroughly. Taste dressing and adjust as desired.

5. Add greens and apples to the dressing. Break the now-cooled pecans apart and add 1/2 of them to the bowl. Gently use your hands to toss the mixture. Top with the rest of the pecans. Divide salad onto six individual plates and serve.

No Salt and Low Salt Dessert Recipes...

26 – Balsamic Grilled Pineapples

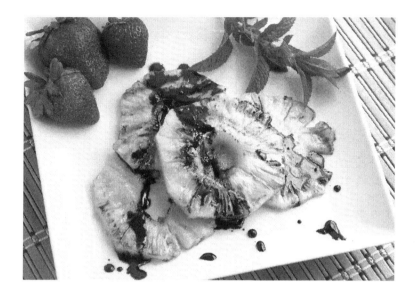

Rich, creamy, no salt added dessert sauce **Makes** this dish special. It is made with honey and yogurt. You can add all kinds of ingredients to the sauce, from vanilla extract to mint, cocoa powder and fruit puree.

Makes 2 Servings

Cooking + Prep Time: 35 minutes

Ingredients:

- 1/4 cup of yogurt, non-fat
- 1 tbsp. of honey, organic if available

- 1/2 tsp. of vanilla extract, pure
- 1 tsp. of vinegar, balsamic
- 8 oz. of pineapple chunks, fresh
- Chopped mint, fresh
- Grapeseed oil spray

Instructions:

1. Combine vinegar, vanilla extract, honey and yogurt in small sized bowl. Whisk well together till fully blended.

2. Preheat oven to 400F. Place non-stick grilling pan inside oven.

3. While oven heats up, place pineapple chunks on skewers. Leave small gaps between chunks.

4. When pan has heated up, sprinkle chopped mint on pineapple. Spray pan lightly using grapeseed oil. Place kabobs in grill pan. Return pan to oven. Cook for five minutes. Turn. Cook for 15 minutes total and turn each five-minute interval. Pour sauce into small sized dishes and serve them beside the skewers.

27 – Banana Peanut Butter Muffins

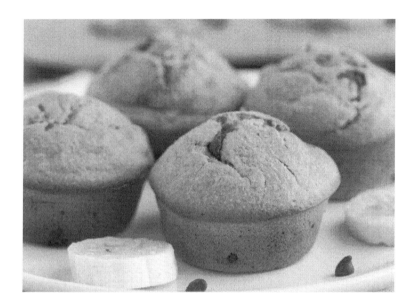

Weekend mornings are even more cheerful when you make these moist, delicious peanut butter and banana muffins. I make it often, if I have ripe bananas I want to use.

Makes 12 Servings

Cooking + Prep Time: 55 minutes

Ingredients:

- 3 ripe bananas, medium
- 1/3 cup of applesauce, unsweetened
- 1 1/4 cups of unbleached flour, all-purpose

- 3/4 tsp. of baking soda
- 1/4 tsp. of salt substitute
- 2 tbsp. of softened butter, unsalted
- 1/3 cup of brown sugar, light
- 2 egg whites, medium
- 1/2 tsp. of vanilla extract, pure
- 10 tbsp. of peanut butter, creamy – divide in 8 tbsp. and 2 tbsp.

Instructions:

1. Preheat the oven to 325F. Use 12 liners to line muffin tin.

2. Mash the bananas in medium bowl and set it aside.

3. Combine salt substitute, flour and baking soda with whisk in medium sized bowl. Set bowl aside.

4. Cream the butter and brown sugar in large sized bowl with electric mixer.

5. Add 8 tbsp. of peanut butter, along with vanilla extract, applesauce, bananas and egg whites. Beat till thickened on med. speed. Scrape sides of bowl down.

6. Add the flour mixture. Blend on low speed till well combined. Don't over-mix.

7. Pour the batter into muffin tins only to halfway full. Add 1/2 tsp. of remaining peanut butter into muffin cups.

8. Top muffins with the rest of the batter. Bake on middle rack for 20-25 minutes, till inserted toothpick comes back clean. Cool a bit and serve.

28 – Mango Sorbet

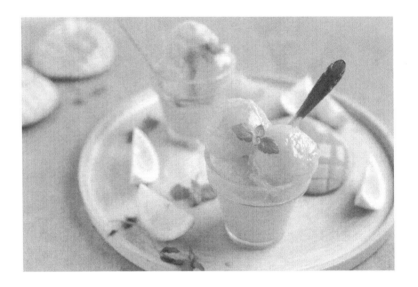

This sorbet can be made with many types of fruit, and the taste is best if the fruit is ripe, but not over-ripe. Two medium sized mangoes are just about the perfect amount for this low sodium treat.

Makes 4 Servings

Cooking + Prep Time: 1 hour 5 minutes

Ingredients:

- 1/2 cup of water, filtered
- 1/3 cup of sugar, granulated
- 2 mangoes, medium

Instructions:

1. Place water and granulated sugar in saucepan on med-high.

2. As water heats up, whisk. When it starts boiling and sugar is dissolving, cook for another one minute as you whisk. Remove from heat.

3. Allow the sugar mixture to cool down for five or six minutes.

4. Peel mangoes. Slice flesh from pits.

5. Place sugar mixture in food processor. Add mangoes. Blend till you have a smooth consistency.

6. Pulse mixture in bursts of 10-seconds each for about a minute.

7. Place mango mixture in plastic container with lid. Place in freezer. Remove and whisk mixture every seven to 10 minutes.

8. As mixture is thickening, use rubber spatula to mix till sorbet has frozen well. Serve.

29 – Quick Apple Phyllo Pie

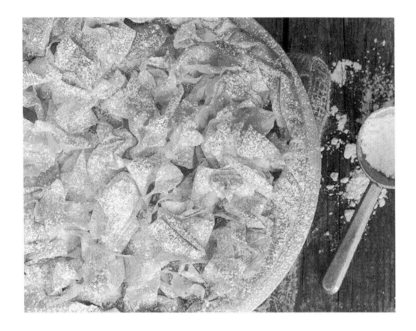

Apple pie is popular, but it usually contains a lot of fat. Not to worry, though – this one doesn't. The phyllo pie crusts make it a low-fat dessert. The best apples to use are Granny Smith, but it works okay with other types, too.

Makes 4 Servings

Cooking + Prep Time: 35 minutes

Ingredients:

- 5 sheets of phyllo pastry
- 38 small oyster crackers, crushed finely (low sodium if you can find them)
- 1 tbsp. of oil, canola
- 1 tbsp. of milk, skim
- 2 apples, large
- 1/4 cup +/- of sugar, granulated
- 2 to 3 tbsp. of corn starch
- Cinnamon, ground
- Sugar, granulated

Instructions:

1. Core the apples, then peel and slice them. Sprinkle with cornstarch and 1/4 cup of sugar. Mix well and set them aside.

2. Mix the milk and oil. Place a sheet of phyllo dough on plate lined with paper towels. Brush the dough with the milk mixture. Sprinkle on 1/4 of crushed crackers. Place another sheet of phyllo on the top. Repeat.

3. Place phyllo sheets in 9" pie pan. Do same with two additional sheets. Place in opposite direction.

4. Fill the pie and sprinkle on cinnamon. Brush last phyllo sheet with the milk mixture, and sprinkle on the rest of the cracker crumbs. Fold it in half. Place atop pie. Fold it over and smooth the edges down on the other phyllo sheets. Brush the top with milk mixture. Sprinkle with the sugar.

5. Bake in 425F oven till browned nicely. Allow to cool a bit and serve.

30 – Raspberry Pears

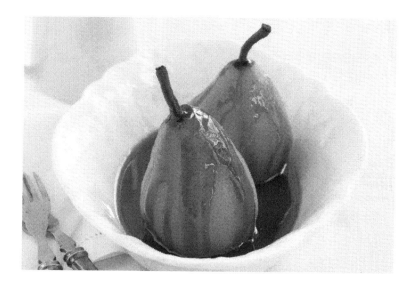

The raspberry sauce weaves its taste into these poached pears, creating a low-fat, special and healthy dessert. It's easy to make and irresistible on the table.

Makes 6 Servings

Cooking + Prep Time: 50 minutes

Ingredients:

- 1/2 cup of spreadable fruit, raspberry, seedless
- 1 cup of juice, apple
- 2 tsp. of lemon peel, grated

- 2 tbsp. of lemon juice, fresh if available
- 3 peeled, quartered Bosc pears, firm

Instructions:

1. Mix all the ingredients except the pears in a 10" skillet. Add the pears.

2. Heat the pan till the mixture boils, then reduce the heat down to med-low.

3. Leave uncovered and simmer for about 1/2 hour. Spoon the juicy mixture over the pears and turn them every 8-10 minutes, till pears become tender. Serve warm, or chill and serve later.

Conclusion

This No Salt added cookbook has shown you...

How to use salt substitutes to create unique tasty dishes both well-known and rare. Modern cuisine does not need excess salt in order to be tasteful.

How can you include it in your home recipes?

You can...

- Make no salt or low salt breakfast dishes, even those that include eggs and potatoes. They are just as tasty as the full-salt meals.
- Learn to cook with salt substitutes, which are widely used in healthy recipes.
- Enjoy making delectable dishes with meats and fish, so you will still be getting your protein and healthy fats. There are SO many ways to make meat and fish dinners without loading up on salt.
- Make dishes using tasty vegetables and fruits, as long as they do not have excessive natural sodium levels.
- Make various types of desserts like fruit sorbets and pies that will tempt your family's sweet tooth.

Have fun experimenting! Enjoy the results!